WEIGHT WATCHERS CROCK-POT SMART POINTS COOKBOOK

Complete Guide Of Weight Watchers Smart Points Slow Cooker Cookbook To Lose Weight Faster And Be Healthier

By James King

© Copyright 2021 -James King -All rights reserved.

In no way is it legal to reproduce, duplicate, or transmit any part of this document by either electronic means or in printed format. Recording of this publication is strictly prohibited, and any storage of this material is not allowed unless with written permission from the publisher. All rights reserved.

Table Of Contents

Introduction..5
   Chapter 1: Why Weight Watchers?...7
   What Is Weight Watcher?...7
   How Weight Watcher Bring About Weight Loss....................................9
   What Is Smartpoints?...10
   How To Calculate Smart Points Everyday You Need?..........................11
   Pros And Cons Of Smart Points...13
   Should I Take More Exercise?..14
   Should I Cut My Foods Intake?..14
   Essential Tips Of Weight Watchers Program.......................................15
   Cautions..16
   FAQs...17
Chapter 2: Why The Crock-pot?...18
   What Is A Crock-pot..18
   Crock-pot vs Other Cooking Appliances..18
   How The Crock-pot Works..19
   Merits Of Using A Crock-pot...19
   Tips For Using The Crock-pot...19
   Different Types Of Crock-pot..20
   How To Choose A Good Crock-pot...21
   Maintenance Of The Crock-pot...21
   FAQs On The Crock-pot(Slow Cooker)..21
Chapter 3: Delicious Slow Cooker Recipes..23
   Recipes Notes..23
   Breakfast & Brunch...23
      1. Egg White Omelet. 24
      2. Bread And Butter Pudding With Marmalade..............................25
      3. Mediterranean Brunch Bake...26
      4. Tapioca-Colanders. 27
      5. Maple and Hazelnut Porridge..28
      6. Sausage Stuffed Peppers..29
      7. Apple Cake..30
      8. Chocolate Rolls. 31
   Lunch & Dinner...32
      1. Potato Casserole..33
      2. Chicken Enchilada Or Tortilla Filling...34
      3. Cheesy Broccoli Casserole..35

4. Collard Greens Cooked In Balsamic...36
5. Rice And Squash..37
6. Pork In Plum Sauce...38
7. Traditional Chili...39
8. Olive And Tomato Chicken..40

Soups & Stews..41
1. Pea Soup..42
2. Sausage Cassoulet..43
3. Chicken And Sprout Bake..44
4. White Bean And Turkey Chili...45
5. Osso Bucco..46
6. Asparagus And Ham Soup...47
7. Provence Stew...48
8. Chicken Noodle Stew...49

Beef, Pork & Lamb...50
1. Mushroom And Beef Meatloaf...51
2. Slow Cooker Bolognese...52
3. Beer Beef Stew..53
4. Bacon Sweet Potato Hash Brown Casserole..................................54
5. Peachy Pulled Pork..55
6. Pork Char Siu..56
7. Lamb Thai Red Curry..57
8. Lamb Rogan Josh..58

Poultry..59
1. Mexican Style Chicken Casserole...60
2. Turkey Bolognese On Zoodles..61
3. BBQ Chicken..62
4. Chicken Carnitas..63
5. Chicken And Broccoli Bake..64
6. Hot And Sweet Turkey...65
7. Buffalo Drumsticks With A Cheese Dip..66
8. Chicken Parmesan Soup..67

Fish & Sea Food..68
1. Shrimp In A Creamy Orange And Chipotle Sauce..........................69
2. Simple Salmon And Potato Bake..70
3. Ginger Shrimp..71
4. White Fish Chilaquiles...72
5. Thai Fish And Pumpkin Soup..73
6. Spicy Mustard Shrimp...74

- 7. Coconut Shrimp Soup..75
- 8. Salmon Laksa..76

Dessert...77
- 1. White Hot Chocolate...78
- 2. Dark Chocolate Mulled Wine Ice Cream Topper.....................79
- 3. Almond, Chocolate And Cherry Kris pies................................80
- 4. Cheesecake...81

Side Dishes..82
- 1. Green Beans And Potatoes With Tomato Salsa.....................83
- 2. Brussels Sprouts, Ham, And Garlic...84
- 3. Bacon Balsamic Green Beans..85
- 4. Caramelized Pineapple...86

Vegan & Vegetarian..87
- 1. Cauliflower Lasagna..88
- 2. Creamed Onion Casserole..89
- 3. Beets And Gnudi...90
- 4. Potato Casserole..91
- 5. Chunky Veggie Chili..92
- 6. Green Bean Casserole...93
- 7. Poblano Corn Chowder...94
- 8. Eggplant Parmesan Bake..95

Beans...96
- 1. Hominy Chili...97
- 2. Santa Fe Black Beans..98
- 3. Chicken And Chickpea Tagine...99
- 4. White Bean And Smoked Ham Soup.....................................100
- 5. Cincinnati Chili...101
- 6. Black Bean And Sweet Potato Chili.......................................102
- 7. White Lime Tofu Chili...103
- 8. Black Bean Soup..104

Conclusion..105

Introduction

Hello friend, this is James King! Welcome to the world of Weight Watchers Program with Crock-Pot cooking. Hope this book will give what you are looking for!

This book will combine Weight Watchers program with Crock-Pot slow cooking, in order to give you a healthy and easy solution about weight loss and overall health, meantime have your favorite delicious recipes. If you are looking for a way to lose weight, if you have no much time to cook foods or aren't familiar with cooking, if you want to know more about Weight Watchers program and Crock-pot cooking, then you should read this book, which will really give you the right answers.

Weight Watchers is not a diet, but a system that guides you and educates you about healthy food and healthy choices in your life. It is based on four essential pillars of weight loss namely *behaviour, food, support and exercise* and it is their constant attention to all four pillars which make the lifestyle successful.

This program is adaptable to different people. No matter you are overweight, obesity or thin, you can have a Weight Watcher program. You can lose weight, increase weight and maintain your weight. Weight Wathcers program don't tell you which food you can eat or can't eat, as it is count in Smart Points, not in calorie, protein, fat or carbohydrate. It is the easiest way of weight loss meantime keep your mouth with flavored foods!

Cooking with a crock-pot is a time-saving, simple and healthy way of cooking. In contrary to the normal cooking methods, you do not need to master a wide range of cooking skills, learn a variety of techniques and spend a lot of time drenching over a hot oven or stove, as the case is always different when using the crock-pot to cook.

In using the crock-pot, everything is often simplified because, you just need to measure and chop your foods for the vast majority of these recipes. And then, for most of them, you won't need anything other than a chopping board, knife, some measuring tools, and your crock-pot.

Also in using this appliance, you no need to worry about what you can or can't have in a student flat or a hotel room, as your crock-pot will do all the work for you. You also no need to worry about putting too much time into it, as you can insert your ingredients together in minutes, leave the house, and come back home in a few hours time to a fully prepared breakfast, lunch, or dinner, I mean life couldn't be more easier.

Combine the Weight Watchers program and Crock-Pot slow cooking really will give you too much convenience. You will like it!

And so in this book, you will learn on how to pick a crock-pot that is right for you, how to use your crock-pot, how to adapt to a new healthy lifestyle and what to cook on different occasions.

Inside this book, we have written 70+ easy and flavored Crock-Pot recipes. All the recipes in this book are detailed with the cooking processes, preparation time, and Smart Points, making it needless of worrying about being rational at calculating calories in ingredients, every time you want to make dinner.

Welcome to the Crock Pot Cooking world! Thanks for your reading!

Chapter 1: Why Weight Watchers?

What Is Weight Watcher?

Weight Watchers is not a diet, but a system that guides you and educates you about healthy food and healthy choices in your life. Whilst Weight Watchers may not be your cup of tea, it is worth exploring and understanding, especially if you intend to use Weight Watchers recipes to lose weight.

Millions of people have lost weight folloing the "Weight Watchers" program. Other diet fads have come and gone, but after 50 years, Weight Watchers is still going strong. Why? Because the program is more than just a diet, it's a lifestyle, which leads to a healthy, happy, balanced individual.

Weight Watchers is based on four essential pillars of weight loss namely

behaviour, food, support and exercise and it is their constant attention to all four pillars which make the lifestyle successful. Their mantra is "the whole person matters" and they approach diet as a core part of the person.

This program is also adaptable to different people. It's no good telling a person who is four hundred pounds overweight to follow the same diet as someone who is close to their ideal weight. The diet would be unrealistic and the overweight person would never be able to follow the diet. They have therefore introduced various eating plans to suit just about every type of person. Weight Watchers also provides one thing which most other diet plans does not - **a huge level of motivation and support**. This is one of the reasons why the program is so successful. Dieting can often be demoralizing and a lonely experience, but with weight watchers you can join a community that knows exactly what you're going through and the leaders of the groups have just the right advice for most people. And if you can't afford to join a group - if you live too far or you don't have the time, then you can join the online community and get the support from the company itself.

The community or groups don't only provide support, but they also add to your sense of accomplishment. The group knows your progress and shares your excitement - even when you've only lost a few ounces - and this sense of accomplishment does wonders for your level of motivation. Because Weight Watchers has been around for so long, there is also tons of information about the diet. Recipes, meal plans and tips are easily found. You can even buy foods with weight watcher points marked on them.

One of the great things about Weight Watchers is the fact that there are no food restrictions. You are not told you can't have something, you are simply told to account for it in your points each day. The problem is, fueling your body with unhealthy options isn't going to give you the result you want.

Yes, you may lose some weight, but your body will still feel sluggish and either hungry or bloated and uncomfortable. Using all points on burgers and fries every day isn't really changing your wellness mentality. You really must work to change the way you look at food and work to feed yourself better options more often than bad. Include some of your favorites on occasion, but focus on healthier things the bulk of the time.

Knowing how to do Weight Watchers for free will save you the expense of monthly meetings that you can turn over and pay for better healthier food options with instead.

How Weight Watcher Bring About Weight Loss

Weight Watchers is a weight loss program that relies on a point system for its recipes and foods, rather than enforcing a specific caloric restriction or other dietary restrictions, to help its followers achieve weight loss. When you follow the Weight Watchers program, you are allowed to eat a certain number of "points" each day. Though some have criticized the program for relying on its own point number system rather than the actual calories, many people have found that it is easier to control how much food they eat when it is presented with an easier point number system like the Weight Watchers' SmartPoints. All food intakes must be controlled at all times, and calories must be accurately calculated. So for this practice to be effective, all members should have a Weight Watchers food scale, or a special kind of calculator that can keep track of your caloric intake.

To make Weight Watchers work, participants share their weight loss goals, eating habits, and activity preferences. The system then generates a daily point average. This average is found by considering how much weight participants want to lose and what the current body weight is. Every day the participants record the foods and quantities that they eat. These foods are assigned point values, and the goal of the participant is to remain within the average points that they are allowed for the day. This teaches participants to eat healthily and to come to an understanding of what they should avoid. For example, a cheeseburger may be 12 points. If a participant only has 20 points total for the day, then eating a cheeseburger will take up over half of their daily points. They can still eat the burger if they would like to, but in order to stick to the diet, they only have 8 points to use for all of the rest of their meals and snacks. But if that person instead had a cup of rice with a side of baked chicken and some spinach, they may only use 7 or 8 points, meaning that they can have more options for other meals. This teaches participants what foods are worse or better than others.

Those who sign up for weight watchers are also given a predetermined number of reserve points they can use whenever they would like. These points can be added to daily totals or can be saved until the end of every week.

What Is Smartpoints?

The SmartPoints plan makes healthy eating simple by putting complex nutritional information into one simple number.   The Smart Points plan is based on the latest in nutritional science, nudging you toward a pattern, not only of weight loss, but of healthier eating with more fruits, vegetables and lean protein, and less sugar and saturated fat. SmartPoints values are generated from the calories, saturated fat, sugars and protein in food. The value is initially determined by the calories, then protein lowers the point value and saturated fat and sugars raise it. The final value is a balance of these factors.

Foods with higher amounts of sugar and saturated fats have higher SmartPoints values. Foods with higher amounts of lean protein have lower SmartPoints values. Many lean proteins like chicken and seafood are now lower in points and sweet treats like muffins, cookies and sugar sweetened beverages are higher. And about 40 percent of foods have stayed the same. Smart Points will still help you lose unwanted pounds, but you may also experience having more energy and seeing your clothes fit better.

A food item can have the same value for calories and protein, but if the sugars or saturated fat are higher in one item versus the other, the point value will be higher. Giving each nutritional item different values in the calculation will help guide you to the healthier food item even though both have the same amount of calories.

How To Calculate Smart Points Everyday You Need?

SmartPoints target is a number based on your gender, Age, Height and Weight.
Gender:
Female- score 2
Male- score 8
A nursing mom- score 12

Age

17-26- score 4

27-37- score 3

38-47- score 2

48-58- score 1

over 58- score 0

Weight

Enter the first one or two digits of your weight in pounds.

(For example, if you weigh 198 pounds, you will add 19 to your score; if you weigh 79 pounds, you will add 7 to your score)

Height

Under 5'1- score 0

5'1-5'10- score 1

Over 5'10- score 2

How do you spend most of your day?

Sitting down? Score 0

Occasional sitting? Score 2

Walking most of the time? Score 4

Doing physically hard work most of the time? Score 6

Just add all of your scores together and that's your daily point allowance.

Now that you know how many points you need to use each day, it's time to figure out what points are in your food. SmartPoints numbers in foods are assigned based on four components. These are calories, saturated fat, sugar, and protein. Protein lowers the amount of SmartPoints values while Sugar and saturated fat increase the SmartPoints values. So, healthier, lower-calorie foods cost fewer points. There is a very accurate calculator for this. Please check [here](#).

As you lose weight, your SmartPoints number adjusts so you can continue to drop pounds. The point number that helps you lose weight initially may be too great when your body shrinks in size. A smaller body uses less energy, so it requires fewer points to continue to lose weight. When you reach your goal weight and switch to maintenance, your Weight Watchers SmartPoints target shifts slightly upwards to keep you from losing too much weight. This higher point value helps even out your energy balance, so you consume and expend relatively equal amounts to maintain your weight. Sustaining a successful weight loss requires you continue to make good food choices most of the time, though.

Pros And Cons Of Smart Points

Pros
- Fruits and vegetables are considered "free foods" which is great for getting yourself to eat more fruits and veggies
- Flexibility to shape your own diet
- Weight loss at a steady rate is more likely to be maintained. But like with any program, consistency makes a big difference.
- Cooking at home is encouraged. You're more likely to eat healthy foods if you cook them yourself.

Cons
- You may need to cut out a lot of your prepackaged snacks and foods (even

ones that are low calorie) as their point value can be way more than they would be if you were just counting calories.
- If you don't like counting calories, you may not like counting SmartPoints either.
- The ability to choose anything you want to eat may prove too tempting for some. It is completely possible to use all your SmartPoints on less-than-nutritious foods. For those dieters, weight loss plans that offer strict eating guidelines may work better.
- You may need to cut out a lot of your prepackaged snacks and foods (even ones that are low calorie) as their point value can be way more than they would be if you were just counting calories.

Should I Take More Exercise?

Although you do not have to exercise to lose weight on Weight Watchers, the program acknowledges the importance of exercise and encourages you to integrate exercise into your weight loss routine. It's great for your health if you eat better and get moving.

Most of us seem to rely on exercise to help us slim down a lot more than we should. That could partly be because we view working out as the cruel tax we have to pay so we can eat that burger we really want.

Should I Cut My Foods Intake?

If you are thinking about reducing your weight the first thing you need to think about doing is lowering your food intake. You know that your weight has increased because you have consumed more food than you actually need and the problem needs to be addressed with some urgency.

The simple solution therefore is to moderate the quantity of food you consume and your weight will disappear. This is in fact true but there is a snag. Simply cutting your food intake can leave you feeling hungry. For the majority of people this feeling of hunger is more than they can tolerate and they begin to let their diet slip. As a result they are unable to lose weight. Not eating is one of the worst things you can do. You will feel physically and emotionally unbalanced. You will crave bad food, your metabolism will slow down and your body will go into starvation mode holding onto fat stores. Eat small amounts and often.

Essential Tips Of Weight Watchers Program

- Keep A Journal - This is a definite must! There is no way to keep track of everything without one. You must update your journal with all the foods/drinks you consume on a daily basis. Most of the times we tend to forget those few snacks that we had throughout the day. By always having your journal handy, write it down immediately whether it be just a few cookies or just a glass of wine.
- Grocery Shopping - Make a list! And before you go grocery shopping, make sure you know the point values of the foods you buy before going to the supermarket. It's a good idea to write down the points values of the items you're going to by next to each item on your list. If something isn't on your list that you found in the supermarket, be sure to read those labels and serving sizes. Calculate those points!
- Use The Calculator - Make some informed decisions and use the SmartPoint calculator to figure out exactly how many points something is

and don't just guess. Knowing how many points something is will help you make that decision if you think you are still hungry and want something more.

- Feel free to mix and match the meals depending on what you fancy.
- If you're hungry, you can snack on fruit and vegetables, which mostly contain 0 Points.
- It's important to drink at least six to eight glasses of fluids throughout the day. This can include coffee, tea, sugar-free squash, diet drinks and water.
- Simply eat three meals a day, and snack on fruit and vegetables which are mostly 0 Points.
- Use snacks with a low point value to prevent hunger throughout the day between meals.
- While you can have anything you want, it's healthier - and will use up fewer points - if you steer clear of typical high-fat, high-sodium snack foods and make nutritious choices.

Cautions

Weight Watchers is not for children under age 10 or pregnant women. Children under age 17 must present written medical permission before they are allowed to partake. Anyone whose weight is within 5 lb (2.3 kg) of the lowest weight should not get on the program. You have to possess a common sense approach on the Weight Watchers program because you can eat what you want to. You could use all your points on chocolate if you want!!! But of course that would not be sensible. You have to be aware of what your body needs as a balance has to be struck. You need protein, calcium, carbohydrates for energy, plus assorted vitamin A and minerals.

Anyone who is under treatment for an illness, taking prescription drugs, or on a therapeutic diet (e.g. low sodium, gluten-free) should consult his/her doctor about the Weight Watchers plan and follow any changes or modifications the physician makes to the Weight.

FAQs

I don't like going to meetings, can't I just do it by myself?
Of course yes! Although the meetings are a huge part of the success but you can get as much success by yourself.

What are some of the best Weight Watcher recipes?
There are a lot of good Weight Watchers recipes out there. You just have to try them out to know which is best for you. Ready to get psyched for some tasty recipes that are easy on your waistline yet satisfying and full of flavor? Check out Weight Watcher recipes.

What advice do you have for someone starting Weight Watchers?
Make the time to plan out your week of food and go grocery shopping at the start of every week. Prep as much as you can in advance, too. If you have trouble with portion control, divide snacks into single portion-sizes in plastic baggies, or buy pre-portioned items.

Is SmartPoint Calculation easy?
Yes, it's easy and gets a lot easier to calculate once you've been on Weight Watcher for a while.

Chapter 2: Why The Crock-pot?

A crock-pot is a unique, innovative cooking appliance that is as significant today as the microwave was in its era. Prior to now, they were outrageously expensive for most people to own, but today, there are many options on the market to suit your budget.

What Is A Crock-pot

A crock-pot is made similarly to a kettle, in that electricity heats up a series of plates and/or tubes to heat the main compartment. Unlike a kettle, the main compartment of a crock-pot is a ceramic pot, which is much like a baking tray, where the ceramic pot is a non-stick that conducts heat very efficiently. It also has a lid to hold in steam, preventing your food from drying out. As heat effective as it is, it cooks meticulously, over a longer period of time than conventional cooking methods. Crock-pots usually have a variety of heat settings, but for the least of it, they come with a dial so you can adjust it to a high, medium, or low. And so for this reason, our recipes will be detailed by those three settings, then due to how the crock-pots multi functionality, it is possible to bake, braise, and stew in it.

Crock-pot vs Other Cooking Appliances

Other cooking appliances are less versatile than the crock-pots because, in using other cooking appliances, you need an entire stove to make a pot of pasta or a whole oven to bake some salmon, a wide range of pots and pans to make all the different foods you want to and so on. However, with a crock-pot you can bake, braise, and stew, and if done carefully you can even fry, all in the same container, as it is small, compacted and portable. Exclusively, the greatest benefit of a crock-pot over other cooking appliances is in the comfortability it presents,when using it. When cooking with other appliances you will always need to be vigilant, so that nothing burns or inflames, and of course in using other appliances, you would not even dare to leave the house with a pot of stew bubbling on the stove top. But with a crock-pot, when used properly, can be left alone to do all the cooking for you. A crock pot is also a very safe way of keeping foods warm where, unlike ovens or microwaves, you can use metallic parts in it.

How The Crock-pot Works

A crock-pot is the combination of an electrically powered heating element and a ceramic bowl. When you switch it on, electricity will slowly heat a series of tubes, like a kettle, or an electric blanket. Thereafter, the tubes will either directly, or through some metal panels, heat a ceramic bowl with your food inside. The lid on the crock-pot prevents moisture, heat leaving and on the other hand, the low temperature preventing any form of burning. With this, we would not be far off from the truth if we concluded that, a crock-pot does the same job as a casserole dish in the oven, except in a much controlled, energy-efficient manner.

Merits Of Using A Crock-pot

There are many advantages to using a crock-pot over other cooking methods, as we discussed earlier in this chapter. But in brief the:

- Crock-pots can be used to cook in a variety of ways.
- Crock-pots cook low and slow, softening your meals to perfection.
- Crock-pots extract all the nutrients from your food and make it easily digestible.
- Crock-pots minimizes prep work and cooking time, requiring little to no attention.
- Crock-pots reduces the number of pots you use to cook a meal, invariably reducing the clean-up time.
- Crock-pots are more energy efficient than using a casserole dish in the oven, but produces similar outcome.
- Crock-pots can be left unattended to, as they cook your meal.
- Crock-pots require no cooking skills beyond knowing how to chop and measure food quantities.
- Crock-pots let you dump all your ingredients into one bowl, and then have a great meal at the end of the day.

Tips For Using The Crock-pot

1. Calculate your timer to the amount of time it will get your food to be done,

if it usually takes 2hours to prepare, then adjust the timer to 2hours.
2. Cook in large portions so that you can refrigerate the meals for future use.
3. Consider buying a divided crock-pot dish to fit your crock-pot, that way you can cook 2-4 different meals at once.
4. Experimentally, crock-pot meals are so versatile, so if you want to try a new ingredient, you can just add it to a meal you think it will work in and then try it out a few hours later.

Different Types Of Crock-pot

There are different types of crock-pot and all of them have their specific purposes. Their specialty are diversified, by so doing causing them to be independently beneficial, where no one is better than the other, no matter than size or brand. It all depends on what you actually want.

- ➔ Basic crock-pots are just made up of a heating element, a ceramic dish, an on-off switch, and a temperature dial. They are perfect for uncomplicated cooking and people on a budget.
- ➔ Timed crock-pots have the added feature that they allow you to decide when your cooking starts and ends. In a pinch, you can use a programmable socket timer instead.
- ➔ Stove-friendly crock-pots: this means you can take the pan out of the crock pot and use it on your stove if need arises.
- ➔ Digital crock-pots can be completely programmed, allowing you to monitor and adjust temperature, time, countdowns, and alarms by single digits.
- ➔ Frying crock-pots, have added functions, like searing, built in so you would not need to undergo any extra steps, like pan-frying or using a stove-friendly crock pot. Certainly a great choice for someone who wants total flexibility.

All crock-pots can also come with a series of attachments to suit your needs. None of these will be used in this recipe book, to make it more accessible to everyone, but you might want to consider:

- ➔ A divider, to allow you cook multiple meals at once.

- → A steamer attachment, so you can steam your food.
- → A lockable lid so you can store and move your meal in the original ceramic pot.

How To Choose A Good Crock-pot

There is no such thing as the "perfect" crock-pot that suit's everyone's needs. When buying a crock-pot, be sure to read the reviews, putting to consideration your location, what you want to cook and how often you will use it. If you're an adult male looking for football boots, you wouldn't get a toddler's first shoes, no matter how good the reviews are, right? So the same is applicable here, look for reviews that mention the things that matter to you like; cooking speed, simplicity, mobility, features, etc.

Maintenance Of The Crock-pot

Maintaining the crock-pot is easy, because the inner part is fully non-stick and many are dishwasher-safe likewise for the lid. So after using your crock-pot, wash the pot, lid and make sure they are completely dry before returning them to the base.

Always check the base for foods that slipped during the process and clean it thoroughly. Also look out for rusts or signs of limescale, as these would in most cases imply that, your crock-pot will need a replacement or repairs.

Make sure that any digital features are accurate, and that it is fitted with a good fuse, especially if you are planning on leaving it on while you are away. Keeping an eye on all electrical components, helps ensure it's proper functionality.

Finally, read the manufacturer's instructions and repair or replace it when it becomes outdated.

FAQs On The Crock-pot(Slow Cooker)

Is it really safe to leave it on?

Yes, slow cookers are designed to be left on for hours at a time, usually up to 10 hours. They use a very low wattage and do not get too hot on the outside. It is perfectly safe to leave a well-maintained slow cooker at home while you are out.

How long can food be kept warm in a slow cooker?

Only use the "warm" or lowest setting in keeping foods that you have cooked. Do not use it to heat up food and do not leave food on "warm" for over four hours.

How can I know my slow cooker is working?

Use a thermometer and make sure your lowest setting (other than "warm") heats two quarts of water to 140F.

What temperature should my slow cooker be?

It should be at least 140F on low and 250F on high.

Can I adapt other recipes for a slow cooker?

Multiply the time by four on high and by ten to twelve on low. That means a fifteen minutes dish should take an hour on high and four hours on low.

Chapter 3: Delicious Slow Cooker Recipes

Recipes Notes

When reading these recipes, please bear in mind the formatting style. At the top of each recipe we will have the name, number of portions, prep time, and cooking time. Under this we will list the smart points of the recipe.

Thereafter, we will list the ingredients measured in cups, ounces and any common allergens will be highlighted in bold. Then we will have the directions, which you should read through before beginning the recipe, to ensure that you are properly equipped with the right tools.

Under each recipe you will find the calories, carbs, protein, and fats per serving, to help make you properly informed. In the nutrition value part: *KCAL for calories; net C for carbs; P for protein; F for fat*.

Breakfast & Brunch

Breakfast is the most important meal of the day and, surprisingly, there are so many ways to make a great breakfast using a crock-pot(slow cooker). Some of the shorter ones are things you can put on as you are preparing in the morning to leave for work or school. Some of the longer ones, are those you can make and refrigerate in the night against the next day. In as much as they are portable, please bear in mind that breakfast foods rarely freezes well.

1. Egg White Omelet.

Yes, you can make an omelet in a slow cooker! If you are eating a high fat diet, consider using 8-10 whole eggs instead of the egg whites.Cauliflower Lasagna.

Serves: 6.
Prep time: 10 minutes.
Cooking: 1h 15 minutes on high.
Smart Points: 3

Ingredients:
- 2 1/2 cups of **egg whites**
- 1 cup of fresh spinach
- 1/2 of cup cherry tomatoes
- 1/2 of cup mushrooms
- 1/4 of cup shredded **cheese**
- Chopped fresh chives
- Pinch of salt and pepper

Directions:
1. Heat your slow cooker up as you prep.
2. Quickly chop all the vegetables ready for mixing.
3. Whisk together the eggs, salt, and pepper.
4. Pour in the vegetables.
5. Pour them into the slow cooker and cover.
6. After 45 minutes, make sure your omelet is completely solid, thereafter add the chives.
7. When it is firm, remove, dice, and serve.

<u>**Nutritional values per serving:**</u> *KCAL: 100; net C 3g; P 13g; F 3.5g. Serve with more fresh chives on top, and sauces.*

2. Bread And Butter Pudding With Marmalade.

Bread and butter pudding is a sort of baked french toast, a staple of English desserts and breakfasts. This version uses up leftover bread that is fast and delightful.

Serves: 12.
Prep time: 15 minutes.
Cooking: 3 hours on high.
Smart Points:8
Ingredients:
- 16 ounces of **bread**, if stale, even better
- 3 tablespoons of **butter**
- 12 ounces of marmalade, or your favorite jam
- 3 cups of **milk**
- 6 whole **eggs**
- 1/3 cup of sugar
- A handful of **walnuts**, crushed or chopped
- Nutmeg, vanilla, cinnamon to taste, or a pudding spice mix

Directions:
1. Slice the bread if it is not already sliced.
2. Butter both sides of the bread and lay the slices in the crock-pot.
3. Whisk the milk, eggs, sugar, and spices together and pour it over the eggs.
4. Leave the eggs to soak up the mix.
5. Cook on high pressure for 3 hours.

<u>*Nutritional values per serving*</u>: *KCAL: 193; net C 16g; P 9g; F 9g.*
Serve topped with the walnuts.

3. Mediterranean Brunch Bake.

This bake makes a great choice for brunches, and you can make it easily in the night before sleeping.

Serves: 10.
Prep time: 20 minutes.
Cooking: 4 hours on low.
Smart Points: 8

Ingredients:
- 8 ounces of sliced **bread**
- 8 **eggs**
- a chopped onion
- 8 ounces of mushrooms
- 14 ounces of broccoli florets
- 1lb plum tomatoes
- 3 ounces of **cheese**
- 1 tablespoon of plain **flour**
- 2 tablespoons of minced garlic
- 2 tablespoons of mustard
- salt and pepper
- 2 tablespoons of herb mix, or ½ tablespoon: oregano, basil, thyme, rosemary

Directions:
1. Toast the bread.
2. Slice the vegetables
3. Place half of the bread slices in the bottom of the crock-pot.
4. Top it with the vegetables and half the cheese.
5. Place the other half of the bread slices on top of the vegetables.
6. Whisk the eggs and seasonings together, then pour in the mix evenly.
7. Sprinkle it with cheese.
8. Cook on a low pressure for 4 hours.

Nutritional values per serving**:** KCAL: 197; net C 16g; P 18g; F 9.5g. Serve as it is.

4. Tapioca-Colanders.

Tapioca can be a nourishing meal to start the day with. Here we go back to its tropical roots and mix it with everyone's favorite tropical mix.

Serves: 8.
Prep time: 15 minutes.
Cooking: 2 hours and 30 minutes on low.
Suitable for: LC, LF, VGI, VGN, PC.
Smart Points: 8

Ingredients:
- ½ a cup of dry tapioca pearls
- 2 cans of **coconut** milk
- ¾ cup of sugar
- 1 egg
- ½ cup of pineapple
- ½ cup of shredded coconut

Directions:
1. Mix the sugar, tapioca, coconut milk and place it in the slow cooker. Cook for two hours.
2. Dice the pineapple finely, or blend it if possible.
3. Combine the egg with a little tapioca and more coconut milk.
4. Add the egg, pineapple, and coconut back to the mix.
5. Wait for 30 minutes before serving.

Nutritional values per serving: KCAL: 150; net C 30g; P 1.5g; F 4g.
Serve topped with pineapple pieces and grated coconut.

5. Maple and Hazelnut Porridge.

Porridge is a breakfast classic that is easy to make in the slow cooker. You could adapt this recipe for any porridge you like.

Serves: 5.
Prep time: 5 minutes.
Cooking: 7 hours on low.
Smart Points: 7

Ingredients:
- 1 cup of oats
- 1.5 cups of **hazelnut milk**
- 1.5 cups of water
- ¼ cup of maple syrup
- ¼ cup of chopped **hazelnuts**
- 2 tablespoons of sugar
- cinnamon and salt to taste

Directions:
1. Mix all the ingredients together in the slow cooker.
2. Cook for 7 hours.

Nutritional values per serving: KCAL: 150; net C 35g; P 7g; F 7g. Serve topped with apples and mixed nuts and seeds.

6. Sausage Stuffed Peppers.

Peppers can make a great meal for any time of day, but the combination of quinoa and sausage makes these ones delectable for brunch.

Serves: 4.
Prep time: 15 minutes.
Cooking: 4 hours on low.
Smart Points: 9
Ingredients:
- 4 bell peppers, your color of choice
- ½ cup dry quinoa
- 4 ounces of sausage meat
- salt and pepper to taste

Directions:
1. Cook the quinoa freshly.
2. Mix the quinoa, sausage meat, and seasoning together.
3. Cut the tops off the peppers, and keep the tops aside, then hollow the peppers.
4. Stuff the peppers with the mix and put the tops back on.
5. Place it in the slow cooker and cook on low for 4 hours.

<u>**Nutritional values per serving**:</u> *KCAL: 100; net C 19g; P 18g; F 13g.*
Serve with a side salad.

7. Apple Cake.

Can you make cake in a slow cooker? Of course you can! This cake is great to produce in advance and store in the fridge if you prefer your breakfast on the go.

Serves: 8.
Prep time: 25 minutes.
Cooking: 1 hour on high.
Smart Points: 8
Ingredients:
- 1.5 cups of   self-raising **flour**
- 1/3 cup of sugar
- 1 cup of applesauce
- 1 cup of apples, chopped
- 1 **egg**
- 1/3 cup of buttermilk or substitute
- salt, cinnamon, nutmeg, and cloves, 1/4 teaspoon each, or 1 teaspoon spice mix

Directions:
1. Line the bottom of the slow cooker with the baking paper.
2. Mix the dry ingredients.
3. Mix the wet ingredients.
4. Mix all the ingredients together and pour them into the crock-pot.
5. Cook on a high for 1.5 hours.

Nutritional values per serving: KCAL: 125; net C 19g; P 4g; F 7g.
Serve topped with more cinnamon and sugar.

8. Chocolate Rolls.

Cinnamon rolls are completely overrated. Just try this chocolate rolls, and I assure you will be a convert. This is another great one for eating on your way to work.

Serves: 14.
Prep time: 20 minutes.
Cooking: 1 hour on high.
Smart Points: 8

Ingredients:
- 2.5 cups of self raising **flour**
- ¼ cup of sugar
- 1 cup of **hazelnut milk**
- 1 cup of hazelnut chocolate spread
- 75g **butter** or margarine
- cinnamon to taste

Directions:
1. Mix all the dry ingredients except for the chocolate spread.
2. Mix all wet ingredients.
3. Stir all ingredients together.
4. Massage the dough.
5. Make strips of the dough, rub one side in the chocolate, and roll them up.
6. Put the rolls in the slow cooker.
7. Cook for an hour on high.

Nutritional values per serving: *KCAL: 188; net C 14g; P 5g; F 15g.*
Serve topped with extra chocolate sauce.

Lunch & Dinner

A good slow-cooker lunch is something you can make lots of in advance and refrigerate or freeze until you wish to eat it, or take it to work. Doing this will save you a lot of time and ensure you are eating healthy no matter what else happens.

A good slow-cooker dinner is something you can prepare the night before or put on in the morning before you go to work, making sure you come home to a fresh, hot, healthy meal.

Therefore, these are the top recipes that take a long time to cook, refrigerate and keep well, and add some healthy variety to your diet.

1. Potato Casserole.

This potato casserole makes a great lunch or light dinner with a salad, but can also make for an excellent side-dish.

Serves: *10.*
Prep time: *25 minutes.*
Cooking: *10 hours on low.*
Smart Points: *7*

Ingredients:
- 30 ounces of potatoes
- 2.5 cups of vegetable broth or bouillon
- 1.5 cups of **fat-free cream** or **cream cheese**
- 5 ounces of **cheese**
- 1 cup of **cornflakes or wheat cereal**
- onion, black pepper, salt, to taste
- chives for topping

Directions:
1. Thinly slice or grate the potatoes down. Thereafter, use the croquettes, hash-browns, or oven fries if you don't want to grate.
2. Pour in all the ingredients in the slow cooker.
3. Cook on a low for 9 hours.
4. Take the lid off and let any remaining liquid cook off in 30-60 minutes more cooking time.

Nutritional values per serving: *KCAL: 134; net C 17g; P 8g; F 6.5g.*
Serve topped with extra cheese and chives, or grilled for a crispy top.

2. Chicken Enchilada Or Tortilla Filling.

Enchiladas, tortillas, nachos, rice... Just pick your easy carb source of choice and assemble on your plate. If you are following a low carb diet, pile this filling high on cauliflower rice or griddled veggies, or just serve in a bowl and enjoy.

Serves: 8.
Prep time: 20 minutes.
Cooking: 6 hours on low.
Smart Points: 8
Ingredients:
- 3 cups of diced chicken
- 3 cans of tomato sauce, you can buy them with herbs already added
- ½ cup of chile
- 1 chopped onion
- 2 cloves of chopped garlic
- 4 chopped red and green peppers
- 1 teaspoon of olive oil

Directions:
1. Heat your slow cooker up with the oil, onions, and garlic and cook for five minutes on high.
2. Turn down to low. Add all over ingredients.
3. Cook for 6 hours on low.

<u>**Nutritional values per serving**</u>: KCAL: 150; net C 15g; P 15g; F 10g. Serve on corn tortillas, beans, rice, veg, etc.

3. Cheesy Broccoli Casserole.

Use dairy substitutes in this delightful casserole dish to make it entirely vegan. The blend of different tastes and textures here makes for a wonderful meal or side dish.

Serves: 6.
Prep time: 20 minutes.
Cooking: 5 hours on low.
Smart Points: 8
Ingredients:
- 2 cups of white rice
- 4 slices of white **bread**
- 4 cups of broccoli tops
- 4.5 ounces of **cheeses** or cheese substitutes
- 2 cups of **milk** or substitute
- ½ cup of **cream** or cream substitute
- 1 onion, chopped
- herb mix and salt to taste

Directions:
1. Combine the rice, cheeses, half the cream and herbs, then hold back a little cheese.
2. Put the oil and onion in the bottom of the slow cooker on a high for five minutes.
3. Mix the other half of the cream, milk, and some salt.
4. Add the broccoli at the base and put the rice mix on top of it, before pouring the cream mix over.
5. Either crumble or place the bread on top. And garnish it with cheese you held back.
6. Cook on low for 6 hours.

Nutritional values per serving: *KCAL: 92; net C 20g; P 16g; F 7.5g.*
Serve with dipping bread.

4. Collard Greens Cooked In Balsamic.

A great side dish or light meal, easy to cook, and very rich and delicious.

Serves: 5.
Prep time: 10 minutes.
Cooking: 6 hours on low.
Smart Points: 7
Ingredients:
- 15 ounces collard greens, chopped
- 1 cup of onion, chopped
- 1 tablespoon minced garlic
- bay leaf
- 3 tablespoons of balsamic vinegar
- 1 tablespoon of honey
- 1 tablespoon of oil
- 2 cups of vegetable bouillon

Directions:
1. Put the onions and oil in the slow cooker on high for five minutes.
2. Add all the other ingredients.
3. Cook on a low for 6 hours.

Nutritional values per serving: KCAL: 82; net C 14g; P 5g; F 2g.
Serve topped with olives and/or cheese.

5. Rice And Squash.

A delightful bake that makes for a good meal or side dish, full of nutritional values.

Serves: 8.
Prep time: 5 minutes.
Cooking: 10 hours on low.
Smart Points: 7

Ingredients:
- 8 cups squash of choice, sliced
- 2 cups boiled of rice
- 1 cup of **cheese**
- 1 cup of **sour cream**
- 2 whisked **eggs**
- ½ cup of bouillon
- ¼ cup of **breadcrumbs**
- salt and pepper to taste

Directions:
1. Mix all the ingredients.
2. Cook on a low for 10 hours.

<u>Nutritional values per serving</u>: *KCAL: 97; net C 14g; P 13g; F 5.5g. Serve with herbs and extra cheese on top.*

6. Pork In Plum Sauce.

With a slight Asian twist, this dish makes for an excellent protein-boosting meal when you are on a low carb diet. You can also reduce the amount of plum sauce, or use a sugar-free plum sauce, for an even lower carb version.

Serves: 8.
Prep time: 5 minutes.
Cooking: 10 hours on low.
Smart Points: 8

Ingredients:
- 2lbs of pork, belly or shoulder work very well for this
- 5 ounces of plum sauce
- 4 plums, chopped and pitted
- 1 cup of bouillon
- 1 tablespoon of allspice
- 1 tablespoon of cinnamon

Directions:
- Make slices in the pork so the flavor soaks through. Then rub it with allspice and cinnamon.
- Mix the remaining ingredients into a sauce.
- Place the pork in crock-pot, and pour the sauce over.
- Cook on a low for 10 hours.

Nutritional values per serving: KCAL: 116; net C 10g; P 14g; F 20g. Serve with a beansprout and raw cabbage salad.

7. Traditional Chili.

This spicy, rich dish full of chocolate, spicy chillies, and beans, will fuel you for days.

Serves: 8.
Prep time: 5 minutes.
Cooking: 8 hours on low.
Smart Points: 8
Ingredients:
- 1.5lbs mince
- 2 cups of diced onion
- 1 cup of diced pepper
- 2 cans of beans
- 2 cans of tomatoes
- 1 cup of bouillon
- 5 chiles
- 2 ounces of dark chocolate
- ½ cup of **sour cream**
- 2 teaspoons of minced garlic
- salt, pepper, cumin to taste, or a chili mix

Directions:
1. Put all the ingredients in a crock-pot and stir well.
2. Cook it for 8 hours on a low.

<u>Nutritional values per serving</u>: *KCAL: 90; net C 15g; P 25g; F 10g.*
Serve with more sour cream and chives.

8. Olive And Tomato Chicken.

A fruity, flavorful slow-cooked chicken suitable for all low carb and whole foods diets.

Serves: 6.
Prep time: 5 minutes.
Cooking: 10 hours on low.
Smart Points: 7
Ingredients:
- 4 lbs of boneless chicken meat
- 2 cans of tomatoes
- ¼ cup of pitted black olives
- 1 teaspoon of olive oil
- 3 teaspoons of paprika
- 1 tablespoon of minced garlic
- salt and pepper to taste

Directions:
1. Put the chicken in the slow cooker.
2. Mix the remaining ingredients together.
3. Pour the sauce over the chicken.
4. Cook on a low for 10 hours.

Nutritional values per serving: *KCAL: 70; net C 9g; P 8g; F 13g. Serve with buttery potatoes and/or broccoli.*

Soups & Stews

Soups and stews are amazingly simple to make in a slow cooker, and will add so much richness and variety to your diet. They are a great way of having a good meal fast, warming on cold days, and delicious. For some of these recipes you will need a blender, but trust me when I say it is all worth it.

1. Pea Soup.

A delightful, low calorie meal for any time of the day. Remove the cream to further reduce calories.

Serves: *6.*
Prep time: *5 minutes.*
Cooking: *5 hours on low.*
Smart Points: *8*
Ingredients:
- 1 chopped red onion
- 4 cups of bouillon
- 2 cups of frozen peas
- ½ cup of **cream** or substitute

Directions:
1. Place all the ingredients in the crock-pot.
2. Cook it for 5 hours on low.
3. Blend.

Nutritional values per serving*: KCAL: 105; net C 15g; P 10g; F 8g. Serve with sour cream or an alternative.*

2. Sausage Cassoulet.

This hearty stew will keep you going all day.

Serves: 8.
Prep time: 10 minutes.
Cooking: 6 hours on low.
Smart Points: 4
Ingredients:
- 1 pound of pork belly
- ½ pound of sausages
- 2 thick rashers of bacon
- 2 cans of beans
- 2 cans of tomatoes
- herb mix
- salt to taste

Directions:
1. Dice the meat.
2. Place all the ingredients in slow cooker and cook on a low for 6 hours.

Nutritional values per serving**:*** *KCAL: 60; net C 14g; P 12g; F 10g. Serve with fresh crusty bread.*

3. Chicken And Sprout Bake.

A nutritious, delicious, low carb meal, and a great way of tricking yourself into eating sprouts, as they are completely smothered and just taste a bit like cabbage.

Serves: 6.
Prep time: 15 minutes.
Cooking: 4 hours on low.
Smart Points: 5
Ingredients:
- 12 ounces of Brussels sprouts, halved
- 12 ounces of chopped boneless chicken
- 1 cup of diced onion
- 16 ounces of mushrooms
- 1.5 cups of **milk** or substitute
- ½ cup of **cream** or substitute
- ¼ cup of **mayo** or substitute
- salt and pepper to taste

Directions:
1. Put all the ingredients in a slow cooker.
2. Cook on low for 4h.

Nutritional values per serving: KCAL: 90; net C 10g; P 15g; F 10g. Serve with cheese on top.

4. White Bean And Turkey Chili.

A healthy twist on a conventional chili that uses white beans and turkey for a low-fat finish.

Serves: 8.
Prep time: 5 minutes.
Cooking: 8 hours on low.
Smart Points: 4
Ingredients:
- 3 cups of turkey mince
- 3 cans of white beans
- 2 cups of diced yellow onion
- 4 cups of chicken broth
- ½ cup of diced tomato, red or green
- 1 tablespoon of minced garlic
- 2 tablespoons of lime juice
- Herb mix including cilantro and oregano
- Salt and pepper to taste

Directions:
1. Mix the ingredients in the crock-pot.
2. Cook for 8 hours on low.

Nutritional values per serving: *KCAL: 86; net C 14g; P 12.5g; F 6g. Serve on a light tortilla with low fat cheese.*

5. Osso Bucco.

This rich, beefy stew is a classic, and a very popular slow-cooker dish to how easily you can get a delicious, restaurant-quality dish.

Serves: 8.
Prep time: 30 minutes.
Cooking: 8 hours on low.
Smart Points: 4
Ingredients:
- 3lbs of bone-in beef
- 2 cups of chopped onion
- 1 cup of chopped celery
- 1 cup of chopped carrot
- 1 tin of chopped tomatoes
- ½ cup of red wine
- 8 chopped garlic cloves
- ¼ ounce of mushrooms
- 1 tablespoon of oil, split in half
- parsley, lemon zest, bay leaf
- salt and pepper

Directions:
1. Put the cooker on high heat with half a tablespoon of oil and the onions.
2. After five minutes, add the remaining oil and the beef.
3. After turning the beef for 10 minutes to brown it a little, add the remaining ingredients.
4. Cover with stock or water and simmer on low for 8 hours.

Nutritional values per serving: KCAL: 86; net C 9g; P 14g; F 6g.
Serve so that every serving has a bone.

6. Asparagus And Ham Soup.

A delicious and rich soup, you can also serve it as a stew if you do not blend it.

Serves: 6.
Prep time: 5 minutes.
Cooking: 4 hours on medium.
Smart Points: 6

Ingredients:
- 2.5 cups of white asparagus
- 1.5 cup of lean ham
- 1 cup of whole milk
- 2 cups of chicken broth
- 2 tablespoons of goat's **cheese**
- Blended herb
- salt and pepper to taste

Directions:
1. Put all the ingredients in the crock-pot.
2. Cook on an average pressure for 4 hours.
3. Blend it.

<u>**Nutritional values per serving**</u>: *KCAL: 147; net C 5g; P 16g; F 7g. Serve dusted with chili powder.*

7. Provence Stew.

A perfect stew for tough cuts of beef, mutton, or goat. The process makes them tender and succulent.

Serves :6.
Prep time: 30 minutes.
Cooking: 8 hours on low.
Smart Points: 9

Ingredients:
- 1.5lbs boneless tough meat, like mutton, chuck roast, hangar, heart, etc
- 1 cup of beef broth
- 2 onions
- 2 cups of carrots
- 3 cups of squash
- 8 garlic cloves
- 2 tablespoons of plain **flour**
- herbes de provence
- salt and pepper

Directions:
1. Roughly dice the meat and vegetables into similarly sized pieces.
2. Put all the ingredients in the crock-pot.
3. Stew it for 8 hours on a low.

Nutritional values per serving: *KCAL: 171; net C 16.5g; P 31g; F 9g. Serve with crusty bread.*

8. Chicken Noodle Stew.

A little heavier and heartier than a chicken noodle soup, this stew is delightful and easy to cook.

Serves: 8.
Prep time: 10 minutes.
Cooking: 4 hours on high.
Smart Points: 6
Ingredients:
- 2 cups of diced chicken breast
- 2 cups of chicken broth
- 2 cups of mushroom or chicken soup
- 1 cup of chopped celery
- 1 cup of chopped pepper
- 1 cup of chopped onion
- 6 portions of dry **spaghetti**
- salt and pepper

Directions:
1. Mix all ingredients other than the pasta into the slow cooker and cook for 3 hours.
2. Add the spaghetti and cook for the remaining hour.
3. Stir and serve.

Nutritional values per serving: *KCAL: 161; net C 18g; P 9g; F 8g.*
Serve with a side salad.

Beef, Pork & Lamb

Red meats are an important part of most people's diets. This is especially true if you're following one of the many options for a low carb diet which are available right now. Red meats do incredibly well in a slow cooker, as the process softens them and melts the fats down, enriching the flavors and textures of the whole dish. Most red meats need to be cooked longer and on a low pressure to give them the most tender texture and get the seasoning to penetrate them. As the crock-pot's lid seals in the evaporated moisture and keeps it condensing and dripping back into the meat, this means slow cookers are an ideal way of making red meat dishes.

1. Mushroom And Beef Meatloaf.

Slow cooker meatloaf is absolutely a thing, that is rich, succulent, and flavorful. This enhanced flavor makes it perfect for adding new and interesting tastes, like wild mushrooms, as they will soak deeply into it.

Serves: 6.
Prep time: 10 minutes.
Cooking: 5 hours on low.
Smart Points: 9

Ingredients:
- 1.5lb of minced beef
- 1.5 cups of diced wild mushrooms
- **2 eggs**
- ½ cup of diced onion
- ¼ cup of minced garlic
- 2 tablespoons of tomato sauce
- 2 teaspoons of mustard
- 1 teaspoon of Italian herbs
- salt and pepper

Directions:
1. Combine the beef, mushrooms, eggs, onion, garlic, herbs, salt and pepper.
2. Form a loaf and place it into a slow cooker.
3. Mix the tomato, mustard, salt and pepper.
4. Spread the tomato and pour it over the loaf.
5. Cook on a low for 5 hours.

<u>***Nutritional values per serving***</u>: *KCAL: 175; net C 5g; P 30g; F 15g.*
Serve with a side salad.

2. Slow Cooker Bolognese.

Bolognese sauce is a great way of making meals in advance. It travels well, chills well, freezes properly, microwaves well, and goes with loads of things, both high and low carb.

Serves: 6.
Prep time: 10 minutes.
Cooking: 8 hours on low.
Smart Points: 9
Ingredients:
- 1lb of ground beef
- ½ lb of ground veal
- 1.5 cups of chopped tomato
- 1.5 cups of chopped onion
- 1 cup of red wine
- 1 cup of beef broth
- ½ cup of chopped celery
- ½ cup of chopped carrot
- 5 minced garlic cloves
- 2 teaspoons of sugar
- 2 tablespoons of Italian herbs
- a bay leaf
- salt, pepper

Directions:
1. Place all the ingredients in the slow cooker.
2. Cook on a low for 8 hours.

<u>Nutritional values per serving</u>: *KCAL: 138; net C 14.5g; P 25g; F 20g. Serve on pasta, or a low carb pasta alternative.*

3. Beer Beef Stew.

There is something about beer and beef that just go together. Beer goes well in many meat dishes, but other than beer and pork, beer and beef are probably the most magical combination.

Serves: *4.*
Prep time: *5 minutes.*
Cooking: *8 hours on low.*
Smart Points: *10*
Ingredients:
- 1lb of boneless, fat-trimmed, diced steak
- 1 can of tomatoes
- 1 cup of diced onion
- ½ cup of beer
- 2 tablespoons of molasses
- herbes de provence
- salt and pepper

Directions:
1. Place all the ingredients in the slow cooker.
2. Cook it for 8 hours.

Nutritional values per serving: *KCAL: 205; net C 20g; P 25.5g; F 8g. Serve with crusty bread, sour cream, or just on its own.*

4. Bacon Sweet Potato Hash Brown Casserole.

This dish works well as a main dish, but if you want to keep your carbs down to a minimum it also makes a nice side dish.

Serves: 6.
Prep time: 10 minutes.
Cooking: 6 hours on low.
Smart Points: 9
Ingredients:
- 6 rashers bacon, chopped and fried
- 32oz grated sweet potatoes
- 1 cup of broth
- 1 cup of chopped onion
- ½ cup of chopped scallions
- ½ cup of **coconut** milk
- salt and pepper

Directions:
1. Combine everything in the slow cooker.
2. Cook it for 6 hours on a low.

Nutritional values per serving: *KCAL: 200; net C 30g; P 12g; F 10g. Serve with a side salad.*

5. Peachy Pulled Pork.

Pulled pork is another fantastic dish to make in the slow cooker. The low temperature renders the fat and relaxes the muscles, giving us juicy and tender meat.

Serves: 12.
Prep time: 30 minutes.
Cooking: 7 hours on low.
Smart Points: 8

Ingredients:
- 3.5lb of pork shoulder, with bone, or ham end, with bone
- ½ cup of chicken stock
- 1 cup of BBQ sauce, homemade or otherwise
- ½ cup of peach jam
- ½ cup of brandy
- pork dry rub

Directions:
1. Mix together the stock, BBQ, jam, and brandy.
2. Slice the top of the pork, add the dry rub, and place the pork in the slow cooker.
3. Pour the sauce over the top.
4. Cook for 7 hours on a low.

Nutritional values per serving: KCAL: 200; net C 18g; P 17g; F 6g.
Serve with fried onions and a side salad.

6. Pork Char Siu.

Char Siu is a long time favourite pork dish of mine, and with this slow cooker recipe it couldn't be any simpler to enjoy it every day at home.

Serves: 8.
Prep time: 5 minutes.
Cooking: 8 hours on low.
Smart Points: 8

Ingredients:
- 2lbs of pork shoulder steak
- ½ cup of vegetable broth
- ¼ cup of **soy** sauce
- ¼ cup of hoisin sauce
- 3 tablespoons of **honey**
- 3 tablespoons of tomato sauce
- 2 teaspoons of minced garlic
- 2 teaspoons of minced ginger
- ½ teaspoon of 5 spice powder

Directions:
1. Mix all the seasonings.
2. Place the pork in slow cooker and pour the sauce on top.
3. Cook it for 8 hours on a low.

<u>Nutritional values per serving</u>: *KCAL: 127; net C 12.7g; P 21.5g; F 9.5g. Serve with a light stir-fry and/or rice.*

7. Lamb Thai Red Curry.

This Thai red curry uses a meat we rarely see on the Thai menus to add extra layers of flavor.

Serves: 8.
Prep time: 5 minutes.
Cooking: 8 hours on low.
Smart Points: 8

Ingredients:
- 2lbs of chopped lamb, lean
- 2 cups of minced onion
- 1 can of **coconut** milk
- 1 cup of vegetable bouillon
- ½ cup of basil leaves
- 4 minced garlic cloves
- 3 tablespoons of red curry paste
- 2 tablespoons of **oyster** sauce
- 2 tablespoons of lime juice
- 1 shredded jalapeno pepper
- salt

Directions:
1. Mix all the ingredients in the slow cooker.
2. Cook on a low pressure for 8 hours.

<u>Nutritional values per serving</u>: *KCAL: 200; net C 10g; P 27.4g; F 5.5g. Serve with jasmine rice or a fresh raw salad.*

8. Lamb Rogan Josh.

This traditional curry is rich, warming, and a lovely meal to come home to. And it takes 8 hours to cook, so you can put it on in the morning and come home to it, all ready for you.

Serves: 6.
Prep time: 15 minutes.
Cooking: 8 hours on medium.
Smart Points: 9
Ingredients:
- 3lbs diced lamb shoulder
- 2 cups of sliced red onion
- 2 tablespoons of Greek **yoghurt**
- 2 tablespoons of **ghee**
- Rogan Josh spice mix
- salt and pepper

Directions:
1. Mix all the ingredient other than the yoghurt.
2. Cook for 8 hours on medium.
3. Serve it with a cool yoghurt on top.

Nutritional values per serving: KCAL: 160; net C 14g; P 38g; F 28g. Serve with yoghurt and rice.

Poultry

Chicken and turkey are the most popular lean meats in the USA, due to their mild, fragrant flavors and delightful texture. Although they can both end up very dry when roasted or fried in the conventional manner, using a slow cooker is a great way to get around this. Thanks to a long, low cook within the sealed crock-pot, moisture gets locked into the bird, ensuring a moist, flavorful meal, where the light and dark meat is cooked evenly. This is also a very safe way of cooking poultry, ensuring it is completely cooked through.

1. Mexican Style Chicken Casserole.

This delicious tortilla-topped casserole is a fairly fast and easy slow cooker recipe which is high in protein and moderate in carbs and fat.

Serves: 8.
Prep time: 15 minutes.
Cooking: 3 hours 30 minutes on high.
Smart Points: 10
Ingredients:
- 2 cups of diced chicken
- 1 can of chicken soup
- 1 can of mushroom soup
- 1 can of chopped tomato
- 1 diced onion
- 1 diced bell pepper
- 10-15 **tortillas**
- 8 ounces of shredded **cheese**
- 1 tablespoon of chili
- 1 tablespoon of garlic
- salt and pepper

Directions:
1. Mix all the ingredients other than the tortillas and cheese together.
2. Crumble the tortillas on top.
3. Cook for it 3 and a half hours on high.
4. Sprinkle it with cheese on top and let it melt.

Nutritional values per serving: KCAL: 182; net C 26.4g; P 21g; F 9.9g. Serve with a side salad or fresh bread.

2. Turkey Bolognese On Zoodles.

If you're looking for a healthy, grain-free, low-carb alternative to the usual weekday night bolognese, you should probably try out this slow cooker turkey bolognese out.

Serves: 4.
Prep time: 15 minutes.
Cooking: 5 hours on low.
Smart Points: 10
Ingredients:
- 1lb of turkey mince
- 1 can of thick tomato paste
- ½ cup of minced onions
- 1 tablespoon of minced garlic
- 2 + 1 tablespoons of olive oil
- 2 teaspoons of sugar
- 3 zucchini
- salt and pepper

Directions:
1. Mix all the ingredients other than the 1 tablespoon of oil and the zucchini into the crock pot.
2. Cook i for 5 hours on a low.
3. Turn the zucchini into a spiral shape.
4. Add olive oil to a pan and heat the zucchini for 2 minutes.
5. Serve.

Nutritional values per serving: *KCAL: 250; net C 26g; P 30g; F 19g. Serve as is, just bolognese on zoodles. Add some cheese if you like.*

3. BBQ Chicken.

If you're looking for something quick and easy to serve for lunch, or to serve at your latest BBQ as the burgers cook, try this.

Serves: 8.
Prep time: 5 minutes.
Cooking: 6 hours on low.
Smart Points: 9

Ingredients:
- 24 ounces of diced lean chicken
- ¾ cup of BBQ
- ¼ cup of **Italian dressing**
- 2 tablespoons of brown sugar
- 2 tablespoons of chicken broth
- 1 tablespoon of Worcestershire sauce

Directions:
1. Mix the sauce.
2. Put the chicken in the slow cooker, and pour the sauce on top of it. Cook it for 6 hours on low.
3. Shred the chicken.

Nutritional values per serving: *KCAL: 166; net C 15g; P 17g; F 3g. Serve on crusty rolls, or tomato boats.*

4. Chicken Carnitas.

Yes, you can make healthy Mexican carnitas in your slow cooker. You just need to focus on the chicken rather than the pork, for a much lower calorie option, and be smart when serving to avoid extra fat and carbs.

Serves: 8.
Prep time: 15 minutes.
Cooking: 8 hours on low.
Smart Points: 8

Ingredients:
- 2lbs of boneless, skinless chicken thighs
- Mexican pulled pork seasoning
- ½ cup of beer
- ½ cup of orange juice
- juice of one lemon
- juice of one lime
- 1 tablespoon of olive oil

Directions:
1. Rub the chicken with the seasoning mix.
2. Put it in the slow cooker, pour the beer and juices on top.
3. Cook for it for 8 hours on a low.
4. Remove and shred.
5. Fry it in a pan with a dash of olive oil to crisp it a bit.

Nutritional values per serving: KCAL: 180; net C 5g; P 29g; F 3g.
Serve as part of a salad bowl.

5. Chicken And Broccoli Bake.

So it definitely isn't the Asian chicken and broccoli you get at authentic restaurants. But it is still a great, healthy combination, and this recipe is tasty and very fast.

Serves: 8.
Prep time: 5 minutes.
Cooking: 8 hours on low.
Smart Points: 8

Ingredients:
- 24 ounces of skinless, boneless diced chicken
- 12 ounces of broccoli florets
- 1 can of evaporated **milk**, low fat
- 1 can of mushroom soup
- ½ cup of low fat **mayo**
- ½ cup of greek **yoghurt**
- ¼ cup of sherry
- ¼ cup of **flour**
- dash of Worcestershire sauce
- salt and pepper

Directions:
1. Mix the liquids and seasonings into a sauce.
2. Put the chicken and broccoli into the slow cooker. Thereafter, pour the sauce on top.
3. Cook it on a low for 8 hours.

Nutritional values per serving: *KCAL: 276; net C 19g; P 21g; F 8g. Serve with rice or salad.*

6. Hot And Sweet Turkey.

The combination of citrus fruits, turkey, and a nice hot sticky sauce, makes this slow cooker dish a delight.

Serves: 8.
Prep time: 5 minutes.
Cooking: 4 hours on low.
Smart Points: 10
Ingredients:
- 4lbs of skinless, boneless turkey thighs, diced small
- 3 cups of diced red onion
- 1 cup of fresh sweet oranges, peeled and chopped
- 1 cup of fresh lemon and grapefruit, peeled and chopped
- 2/3 cup of fresh orange juice
- 1/3 cup of sugar-free marmalade
- 2 teaspoons of tamarind paste
- 2 teaspoons of 5 spices
- salt and pepper

Directions:
1. Combine all ingredients in the slow cooker.
2. Cook it on a low for 4 hours.

Nutritional values per serving: KCAL: 277; net C g25; P 29g; F 6g.
Serve with corn bread.

7. Buffalo Drumsticks With A Cheese Dip.

A great hot spicy kick, and a low calorie snack meal, for you, when you need a light meal packed with flavor. Calories of course vary depending on what dip you use, and how much of it.

Serves: 8.
Prep time: 10 minutes.
Cooking: 3 hours on high.
Smart Points: 4

Ingredients:
- 1.5lbs of skinned chicken drumsticks
- ½ cup of buffalo sauce
- salt and pepper
- **cheese** dip

Directions:
1. Dip the drumsticks in the sauce so they get coated properly.
2. Put the drumsticks in the slow cooker and pour the remaining sauce on top.
3. Cook on a high for 3 hours.

Nutritional values per serving: *KCAL: 95; net C 4.5g; P 8g; F 5g.*
Serve with veggie sticks.

8. Chicken Parmesan Soup.

This works as a lovely alternative to the traditional chicken noodle soup.

Serves: 6.
Prep time: 5 minutes.
Cooking: 4 hours on high.
Smart Points: 8

Ingredients:
- 1.5lbs of boneless, skinless chicken breast
- 3 cups of chicken broth
- 1 can of chopped tomatoes
- 6 ounces of dry shaped **pasta**
- ½ cup of Parmesan **cheese**
- 1 red bell pepper, diced
- 1 zucchini, diced
- ½ an onion, diced
- salt and pepper

Directions:
1. Put all the ingredients except the pasta in the slow cooker and cook on a high for 3 hours 30 minutes.
2. Add the pasta, and cook for another 10-30 minutes.

Nutritional values per serving: *KCAL: 145; net C 23g; P 27g; F 5g.*
Serve with extra Parmesan on top.

Fish & Sea Food

Fish and sea food are amazing sources of protein, vitamins, and minerals. This is because the healthiest people on our planet are pescetarians, and swapping your red meats for fish could add over a decade to your life span. But despite its health benefits, for many people fish can seem a little too... nasty. And if you don't have experience cooking it, you may not be sure where to even start. These recipes were therefore chosen with the everyday man in mind. They are delicious, simple to cook, not too fishy, and perfectly suited to a pescetarian or omnivorous diet. You will be focusing on shrimp, salmon, and white fish, as these fish have many benefits, but are also good at taking on flavors around them, making it easy for fish lovers and non-fish-lovers to both enjoy these dishes.

1. Shrimp In A Creamy Orange And Chipotle Sauce.

This is an insanely fast shrimp recipe that will give you stacks of protein in the time, as you get changed from work, have a shower, and set the table

Serves: 4.
Prep time: 5 minutes.
Cooking: 1 hour on high.
Smart Points: 7
Ingredients:
- 1.5lbs of peeled and defined **shrimp**
- 2/3 cup of half and half
- 1 chipotle chile
- 1 teaspoon of orange zest
- salt and pepper

Directions:
1. Blend the half, chile, orange, salt, and pepper.
2. Put in the crock-pot with the shrimp, and cook for 1 hour on high.

Nutritional values per serving: KCAL: 186; net C 3g; P 28g; F 6g.
Serve on top of rice, noodles, or salad.

2. Simple Salmon And Potato Bake.

Salmon is one of the best fish for us, and has a distinctive creamy non-fishy taste which many will appreciate.

Serves: 4.
Prep time: 5 minutes.
Cooking: 2 hours on low.
Smart Points: 8

Ingredients:
- 4 **salmon** fillets
- 2 ounces of baby potatoes
- 1 ounce of cherry tomatoes
- 1 lemon, halved
- 2 tablespoons of thyme
- salt and pepper

Directions:
1. Rub the salmon with the salt, pepper, lemon juice, and thyme.
2. Place it in the slow cooker with potatoes, tomatoes, and a little water, around half an inch.
3. Cook on a low for 2hours.

Nutritional values per serving: *KCAL: 167; net C 11g; P 37g; F 22g. Serve with green beans, wilted spinach, or salad.*

3. Ginger Shrimp.

One of the biggest benefits of cooking with shrimp is that it soaks up any flavor around it. This ginger shrimp is tangy and delicious.

Serves: 4.
Prep time: 5 minutes.
Cooking: 1 hour on low.
Smart Points: 5

Ingredients:
- 1lb of peeled and deveined **shrimp**
- 1 cup of minced onion
- 1 cup of minced garlic
- ½ cup of water
- 1 tablespoon of sake or mirin
- 2 teaspoons of **soy** sauce
- 2 teaspoons of **corn** starch
- 1 teaspoon of fresh ginger, grated
- 1 teaspoon of sugar
- 1 teaspoon of **sesame seeds**
- salt and pepper

Directions:
1. Mix the sauce.
2. Add the shrimp.
3. Put it in the slow cooker and cook for an hour on low pressure.

Nutritional values per serving: KCAL: 192; net C 7g; P 24g; F 7g.
Serve with salad.

4. White Fish Chilaquiles.

Everywhere has a white fish that is cheap to buy, really plain tasting, and low in fat and calories. For us it is Pollock and basa, but for you it may be something else. The mild taste and meaty, flaky texture of these fish makes them a perfect substitute for chicken in dishes like chilaquiles.

Serves: 10.
Prep time: 15 minutes.
Cooking: 4 hours on low.
Smart Points: 9

Ingredients:
- 2.5lbs of boneless white **fish**, cubed
- 5 cups of **tortilla chips**
- 2 cans of diced tomatoes
- 2 cups of chopped mixed bell peppers
- 1.5 cups chopped red onion
- 1 cup of chopped chiles
- ¾ cup of bouillon
- 2/3 cup of **queso fresco, or cottage cheese**
- ¼ cup of cilantro

Directions:
1. Mix all ingredients except the tortilla chips and cheese, into the slow cooker.
2. Cook on a low for 4 hours.
3. Place the tortilla chips on top and crumble the cheese all over.

<u>**Nutritional values per serving:**</u> *KCAL: 219; net C 23g; P g25; F 2.5g. Serve with a side salad and more cilantro for garnish.*

5. Thai Fish And Pumpkin Soup.

This warming, hearty soup can be left on a low all day, until you're ready to come home and enjoy it's comforting, creamy goodness.

Serves: 4.
Prep time: 30 minutes.
Cooking: 8 hours on low.
Smart Points: 9
Ingredients:
- 1.5lbs of chunky white **fish**
- 3 cups of bouillon
- ½lb of pumpkin puree
- ½ tin of **coconut** milk
- Thai red curry paste

Directions:
1. Mix the sauce.
2. Put the fish in the crock-pot and pour the sauce over it.
3. Cook on a low for 8 hours.

Nutritional values per serving: *KCAL: 235; net C 22g; P 37g; F 12g. Serve over jasmine rice.*

6. Spicy Mustard Shrimp.

If you want shrimp with some real bite, try out this quick and easy recipe for mustard shrimp.

Serves: 4.
Prep time: 10 minutes.
Cooking: 1 hour on high.
Smart Points: 8
Ingredients:
- 1lb of peeled and deveined **shrimp**
- 1 cup of mango puree
- 1 cup of diced green onion
- ¼ cup of cilantro
- 1 tablespoon of mustard
- 1 tablespoon of hot sauce
- 1 tablespoon of lime juice

Directions:
1. Mix all the ingredients together in the slow cooker.
2. Cook on a high for an hour.

<u>Nutritional values per serving</u>: *KCAL: 181; net C 10g; P 23g; F 4.5g. Serve with rice or fried green vegetables.*

7. Coconut Shrimp Soup.

If you are fancying something rich, creamy, and coconutty, this is a perfect time to try out our coconut shrimp soup.

Serves: *4.*
Prep time: *5 minutes.*
Cooking: *1 hour on high.*
Smart Points: *8*

Ingredients:
- 1lb of peeled and deveined **shrimp**
- 1.5 cup of bouillon
- 1 can of **coconut** milk
- 1 cup of diced red and yellow bell peppers
- 1 tablespoon of **fish** sauce
- 1 tablespoon of lime juice

Directions:
1. Mix all the ingredients.
2. Cook for an hour on high pressure.

Nutritional values per serving: *KCAL: 185; net C 12.5g; P 22g; F 6g. Serve with a scoop of jasmine rice or cauliflower rice at the bottom of the bowl.*

8. Salmon Laksa.

This warming salmon dish is a great way to eat some healthy oily fish.

Serves: 4.
Prep time: 5 minutes.
Cooking: 4 hours on low.
Smart Points: 8
Ingredients:
- 4 **salmon** fillets
- 1 can of **coconut** milk
- 1 cup of bouillon
- 1 zucchini, finely sliced
- 1 cup of bean sprouts
- 200g **vermicelli**
- a jar of laksa paste

Directions:
1. Mix all the ingredients except the vermicelli.
2. Cook on a low pressure for 4 hours.
3. Quickly Blanche the vermicelli.
4. Serve.

Nutritional values per serving: *KCAL: 120; net C 24g; P 26g; F 29g. Serve in a bowl, to ensure plenty of broth is there.*

Dessert

Desserts may be something you usually buy, but if you want a delicious treat, there are several gorgeous recipes which you can make in your slow cooker. They're all pretty quick and simple if preserved well in the fridge. To boot, you can break the recipes down into smaller batches if you want them to last you longer. None of these are health foods, technically speaking, but some are suitable if you're on a diet, some can be adapted to suit your diet, and all are delicious.

1. White Hot Chocolate.

Hot chocolate is always delicious, while this type is always even more better. It makes a wonderful warming pudding or treat on a cold day.

Serves: 8.
Prep time: 10 minutes.
Cooking: 30 minutes on high.
Smart Points: 8
Ingredients:
- 2 pints of **milk**
- 2 pints of **cream**
- 4 ounces of white chocolate
- 1 teaspoon of nutmeg

Directions:
1. Melt all the ingredients in the slow cooker, stirring continually.
2. Serve as soon it is blended properly.

Nutritional values per serving: KCAL: 170; net C 27g; P 11g; F 26.5g. *Serve dusted with cocoa powder.*

2. Dark Chocolate Mulled Wine Ice Cream Topper.

Not exactly a dessert, but an amazing addition to one. With this topper, even plain frozen yoghurt or simple fruit will be elevated.

Serves: 10+.
Prep time: 5 minutes.
Cooking: 1 hour on low.
Smart Points: 4
Ingredients:
- 1 cup of red wine
- 2 ounces of dark chocolate
- ½ cup of sugar
- ½ cup of corn syrup
- 1/3 cup of cocoa powder

Directions:
1. Put the wine in the slow cooker on a low, with the lid off, for 1 hour.
2. Add the other ingredients, stirring until it is combined.
3. Refrigerate it until needed.

Nutritional values per serving: *KCAL: 80; net C17 g; P 0g; F 1g.*
Serve on top of any and every conceivable dessert.

3. Almond, Chocolate And Cherry Kris pies.

An incredibly fast recipe for an adult take on his/her childhood's favorite. This recipe is rich, delicious   and these they will last you for a week.

Serves: 36.
Prep time: 5 minutes.
Cooking: 30 minutes on low.
Smart Points: 2
Ingredients:
- 1 cup of semisweet chocolate
- 1 cup of white chocolate
- 1.5 cup of **rice** cereal
- ¾ cup of dried cherries
- 1/3 cup of **almond** flour

Directions:
1. Warm the chocolate, stirring continually, until it is melted.
2. Turn off the slow cooker and stir in the almond flour.
3. Wait a bit, then add the dried cherries.
4. Wait a bit longer, then add the rice cereal.
5. Make the 36 little flat Kris pies and refrigerate it.

<u>Nutritional values per serving</u>: *KCAL: 68; net C 7g; P 0g; F 3.3g. Serve out of your hand. It's a snack, after all.*

4. Cheesecake.

Yes, a slow cooker cheesecake! This recipe leaves you with a gorgeous, silky cheesecake that you can put that wine and chocolate sauce on.

Serves: 10.
Prep time: 20 minutes.
Cooking: 2 hours on high.
Smart Points: 7
Ingredients:
- 2/3 cup of crumbled **cookies**
- 2 tablespoons of melted **butter**
- 1 tablespoon of icing sugar
- 24 ounces of low fat cream **cheese**
- 2/3 cup of white sugar
- 2 **eggs**
- 1 tablespoon of **flour**
- jam

Directions:
1. Place the base of metal pan with a baking paper.
2. Mix the cookies, butter, and sugar.
3. Push the mixture into the bottom of the pan.
4. Blend the cheese, sugar, eggs, and flour.
5. Pour on it top of base.
6. Pour a cup of hot water into the crock pot.
7. Make a foil ring and place it in the water.
8. Rest the metal pan on top of the ring.
9. Cook it for 2 hours on a high.
10. Refrigerate.

Nutritional values per serving: *KCAL: 232; net C 22g; P 11g; F 24g. Serve with a drizzle of jam.*

Side Dishes

A good side dish or two are essential to eating and living well. They add color and texture to our meal, make our plates look great, stop us from eating fries in every meal, and impress our guests when they are around. What is more, a tasty side dish makes a great meal when you don't have much time, or have overeaten. These slow cooker recipes make it easy to master four delicious side dish recipes. And all of them can be made in advance and reheated in time to accompany the main course, so there's no need to worry if you need your slow cooker for both.

1. Green Beans And Potatoes With Tomato Salsa.

A wonderful vegetable based side dish full of texture, complementary flavors and acid-alkaline balance.

Serves: 8.
Prep time: *5 minutes.*
Cooking: *2 hours on high.*
Smart Points: *4*
Ingredients:
- 1lb green of beans, trimmed
- 1lb of tomato, chopped
- 1.5 cup of diced potato
- ½ cup of celery
- ¼ cup of water
- 1 tablespoon of olive oil
- 1 tablespoon of minced garlic
- salt and pepper

Directions:
1. Put the potatoes and beans in the pot with the water. Cook on a low for one hour.
2. Add the remaining ingredients, toss and then cook on a low for another hour.

<u>**Nutritional values per serving**</u>: *KCAL: 70; net C 11g; P 2g; F 3g.*
Serve with juicy or saucy protein dishes.

2. Brussels Sprouts, Ham, And Garlic.

If you want to enjoy sprouts, you need to cook them through, but not letting them go mushy, and season them well. You can achieve this using the high heat setting of a slow cooker.

Serves: 12.
Prep time: 10 minutes.
Cooking: 2 hours on high.
Smart Points: 4

Ingredients:
- 3lbs of Brussels sprouts
- ¼ cup of diced ham
- 1 slice of white **bread**
- 3 minced garlic cloves
- 2 tablespoons of lemon juice
- salt and pepper

Directions:
1. Mix all the ingredients except the bread together.
2. Cook on a high for 2 hours.
3. Crumble the bread on top and process it in a hot oven for five minutes.

Nutritional values per serving: *KCAL: 58; net C 9.5g; P 4.5g; F 1g. Serve with sweet or mild tasting dishes.*

3. Bacon Balsamic Green Beans.

Another variant on green beans, this side dish is less sweeter than the first one, much tangier and saltier.

Serves: 8.
Prep time: *5 minutes.*
Cooking: *2 hours on low.*
Smart Points: *5*
Ingredients:
- 2lbs of green beans
- 1lb of bacon
- ¼ cup of minced shallots
- ¼ cup of balsamic vinegar

Directions:
1. Mix all the ingredients together in slow cooker.
2. Cook for 2 hours on a low pressure.

<u>Nutritional values per serving</u>: *KCAL: 192; net C 12g; P 18g; F 8g. Serve with high carb dishes, or alongside large salads.*

4. Caramelized Pineapple.

Pineapple is often used to add acidity, but when you caramelize it you kill that acidity and take the sweetness out. This makes for a very versatile side dish.

Serves: 4.
Prep time: 15 minutes.
Cooking: 2 hours on high.
Smart Points: 4

Ingredients:
- 2 cups of diced pineapple
- 1 tablespoon of **soy** sauce
- 1 tablespoon of minced garlic
- 1 tablespoon of minced sweet Spanish onion
- 1 teaspoon of chili powder
- 1 teaspoon of cilantro
- 1 teaspoon of grated ginger
- 1 teaspoon of oil

Directions:
1. Mix everything except for the pineapple and the oil.
2. Pat the pineapple dry and roll it in the mixture.
3. Put the oil in the base of the slow cooker and put it on high.
4. When the oil is hot, add the pineapple and cove it.
5. Return to stir every 30 minutes, alternatively, make sure a bit of every pineapple cube is touching the base or sides and just let it cook for 2 hours.

<u>*Nutritional values per serving*</u>: *KCAL: 61; net C 11g; P 1g; F 2g.*
Serve with dry proteins, hot foods, and salty foods.

Vegan & Vegetarian

Following a vegan or vegetarian diet can be difficult in the first place, as more foods have animal products than a non-vegan or non-vegetarian would ever suspect. This is especially true of healthy food, tasty food, and quick meals, where combining them seems almost impossible. It always seems like a case of "pick 2", where your food could be healthy, tasty and time-consuming. But with your slow cooker you will be able to cook amazing, delicious, healthy vegan and vegetarian meals in no time at all. Whether you are a seasoned veteran who is just looking for more ideas, or a newbie who has no idea how to eat a healthy vegan or vegetarian diet, a slow cooker can be your friend, introducing new, interesting methods and flavors to your cooking plans. Most of these recipes can be made vegan by using dairy supplements.

And don't forget: all the recipes in this book can be made vegan or vegetarian if you swap in the vegan mince for the beef and the firm tofu for white meats and fish.

1. Cauliflower Lasagna.

Cauliflower cheese is a long-time household favorite, especially for vegetarians. And with the development of more advanced vegan cheeses which melts and lightly caramelizes, now these dishes are even better for people eating dairy-free.

Serves: 6.
Prep time: 20 minutes.
Cooking: 4 hours on high.
Smart Points: 4
Ingredients:
- 2lbs of cauliflower, sliced ½ inch thick
- 8 **lasagna sheets**
- 3 cups of **milk** or alternative
- 1.5 cup of **cheddar** or alternative
- ½ cup of **Parmesan** or alternative
- ¼ cup of **breadcrumbs**
- ¼ cup of **flour**
- 1 tablespoon of **butter** or any other alternative
- Herb mix
- salt and pepper

Directions:
1. Warm the milk and pour in the cheeses, crumbs, flour, herbs, salt and pepper. Reserve a handful of the cheese.
2. Melt the butter and brush the cauliflower slices on both sides with it.
3. Put grease proof paper to line your crock-pot.
4. Place the cauliflower, lasagna sheets, and cheese.
5. Top it with the remaining cheese.
6. Cook on high pressure for 4 hours.

Nutritional values per serving: KCAL: 124; net C 26g; P 15g; F 5g.
Serve with crusty garlic bread.

2. Creamed Onion Casserole.

This casserole is perfect for everyone whose favorite part of a veggie dog is the fried onion, and who adores French onion soup.

Serves: 8.
Prep time: 35 minutes.
Cooking: 9 hours 30 minutes on low.
Smart Points: 6

Ingredients:
- 4 cups of thinly sliced leeks
- 3 cups of thinly sliced onion
- 2 cups of **milk** or alternative
- ½ cup of white wine
- ¼ cup of **flour**
- ¼ cup of **breadcrumbs**
- 2 tablespoons of olive oil
- Herb mix
- salt and pepper

Directions:
1. Reduce the white wine to half by simmering it.
2. Make a white sauce with the oil, flour, milk, salt and pepper.
3. Mix the wine, sauce, and all remaining ingredients except the breadcrumbs together and hold back some herbs. Pour them into the crock-pot.
4. Sprinkle the breadcrumbs and the remaining herbs on top.
5. Cook on a low for 9 and a half hours.

Nutritional values per serving: KCAL: 156; net C 25g; P 5g; F 4g.
Serve with crusty bread and a side salad.

3. Beets And Gnudi.

Gnudi? What's a gnudi? Well, a gnudi is a soft cheese and flour dumpling, a little like an inverted gnocchi, and they are greatly delightful.

Serves: 4.
Prep time: 25 minutes.
Cooking: 3 hours on low.
Smart Points: 8

Ingredients:
- 1lb of fresh golden beetroot
- 1lb of fresh semi-hard or soft **cheese**, or alternative
- 100g of chopped **butter** or alternative
- 2/3 cup of plain **flour**
- ½ cup of **Parmesan** or alternative
- 1 tablespoon of minced garlic
- 1 tablespoon of lemon juice
- Herb mix
- salt and pepper

Directions:
1. Gently fold the butter into the flour until the crumbs are formed.
2. Pour in the cheese, herbs, salt and pepper.
3. Mix the lemon, garlic and toss the gnudi in it.
4. Put a cup of water in your slow cooker and add a foil doughnut.
5. Put the gnudi on a pan and put it in the slow cooker.
6. Cook it on a low for 3 hours.
7. Spiralize the golden beetroot and toss it into the Parmesan, salt, and pepper.
8. Serve the gnudi on the surface of the fresh beetroot slaw.

<u>Nutritional values per serving</u>: *KCAL: 191; net C 22g; P 16.9g; F 27g. Serve as is, or with more parmesan for sprinkling.*

4. Potato Casserole.

This casserole uses your usual frozen hash browns in a new and creative way to make a tasty dinner, or side dish.

Serves: 10.
Prep time: 25 minutes.
Cooking: 12 hours on low.
Smart Points: 8

Ingredients:
- 32 ounces of hash browns
- 3 cups of **cornflakes**
- 1.5 cup of **milk** or alternative
- 1 cup of chopped onion
- 1 cup of chopped bell pepper
- 2/3 cup of **yoghurt** or alternative
- 4 ounces of **cheddar** or alternative
- 2 tablespoons of melted **butter** or alternative
- salt and pepper

Directions:
1. Defrost and mash the hash browns.
2. Mix the flour and butter well, then add the warm milk and mix it to make a white sauce.
3. Add the seasonings, yoghurt and cheese to the mixture, and fold in the onions and bell pepper.
4. Quickly pour in the hash browns and scoop it into the slow cooker.
5. Disintegrate the cornflakes on top.
6. Cook it for 12 hours on a low.

<u>**Nutritional values per serving**</u>: *KCAL: 235; net C 32g; P 9g; F 8g.*
Serve with a side salad, or as a side to a protein-heavy meal.

5. Chunky Veggie Chili.

Everyone needs a good, simple, fast and a delicious chili recipe, whether vegan or not.

Serves: 8.
Prep time: 10 minutes.
Cooking: 8 hours on low.
Smart Points: 8

Ingredients:
- 2 cups of chopped onions
- 2 cups of chopped peppers
- 2 cans of chopped tomatoes
- 2 cans of black beans
- 1 can of kidney beans
- 1 can of pinto beans
- 4 squares of dark chocolate
- 1 tablespoon of minced garlic
- 1 tablespoon of brown sugar
- 1 tablespoon of chili powder
- 1 teaspoon of cumin
- 1 teaspoon of oregano
- salt and pepper

Directions:
1. Place all ingredients in the crock pot.
2. Cook it on a low for 8 hours.

Nutritional values per serving: *KCAL: 257; net C 39g; P 13g; F 2.5g. Serve with crusty bread or corn bread and avocado.*

6. Green Bean Casserole.

Even green beans, cooked correctly, can make for a hearty meal that is also healthy for you and incredibly easy to make.

Serves: 8.
Prep time: 25 minutes.
Cooking: 10 hours on low.
Smart Points: 5
Ingredients:
- 1.5lbs of trimmed green beans
- 8 ounces of mushrooms
- 1.5 cup of **milk** or alternative
- 1 cup of deep fried onions
- ½ cup of **breadcrumbs**
- ½ cup of **buttermilk** or alternative
- ¼ cup of **flour**
- 2 tablespoons of **butter** or alternative
- 1 tablespoon of **ranch** dressing
- Herb mix
- salt and pepper

Directions:
1. Combine the butter and flour.
2. Dissolve it into the warm milk.
3. Mix all ingredients except for the breadcrumbs and onions.
4. Put it in a slow cooker and top it with breadcrumbs and onions.
5. Cook for 10 hours on a low.

<u>Nutritional values per serving</u>: *KCAL: 168; net C 18.5g; P 6g; F 8g.*
Serve with crusty bread or an orange and red onion salad.

7. Poblano Corn Chowder.

This recipe is brilliant for a warm and comforting slow cooker meal.

Serves: 8.
Prep time: 5 minutes.
Cooking: 8 hours on low.
Smart Points: 6
Ingredients:
- 2 cups of fresh **corn**
- 1 can of creamed **corn**
- ½ cup of **milk** or alternative
- 2 large **eggs**
- 4 ounces of **cheddar** or alternative
- 4 poblano chiles
- 2 tablespoons of sugar
- salt and pepper

Directions:
1. Beat the eggs.
2. Mix all the ingredients in the slow cooker.
3. Cook for 8 hours on a low.

Nutritional values per serving: *KCAL: 183; net C 26g; P 9g; F 6g. Serve with crusty bread or nachos.*

8. Eggplant Parmesan Bake.

This dish is a delicious, tangy, and a low fat, but still high in flavor. This makes it a perfect meal for the middle of the week, or a light weekend lunch.

Serves: 8.
Prep time: 30 minutes.
Cooking: 8 hours on low.
Smart Points: 8

Ingredients:
- 2lbs of sliced eggplant
- 3 cups of **mozzarella** or alternative
- 4 cans of tomato sauce
- 2 cans of chopped tomatoes
- 1 can of tomato paste
- 1.5 cups of **breadcrumbs**
- ½ cup of white wine
- ¼ cup of water
- ¼ cup of **Parmesan** or alternative
- 3 **egg whites**
- 1 tablespoon of minced garlic
- Herb mix
- salt and pepper

Directions:
1. Salt the eggplants and leave.
2. Beat the egg whites and add the water.
3. Mix the breadcrumbs and Parmesan.
4. Pat the eggplants dry and dip it first in egg then in Parmesan.
5. Fry the eggplants, because the hotter the better. Deep fry if you can.
6. Mix all the remaining ingredients.
7. Place the eggplants and sauce in a slow cooker.
8. Cook it on a low for 8 hours.

<u>**Nutritional values per serving**</u>: *KCAL: 198; net C 28.5g; P 20g; F 8.5g. Serve with a side salad or ratatouille.*

Beans

Beans are the alternative protein choice for many people around the world. They have a great combination of carbs and proteins with minimal fats, that are completely plant based, loaded with fibre, and rich in vitamins and minerals. The only problem is, to an inexperienced person beans may seem boring, or like an insurmountable challenge. We are all, only familiar with beans as a side dish, or an annoying intrusion in our meals. But outside of the USA, the UK, and Canada, beans are actually a core part of many traditional diets. Most cultures around the world would gladly chow down on a bowl of beans for lunch. Why? Are their beans much different to ours? No, it's just that they're cooking them right. A slow cooker is a great way to make the most of beans, letting you cook them even from dry without it taking much effort. Just follow these recipes, and you will be eating tasty beans in no time.

1. Hominy Chili.

Hominy, for those who do not know, is a dried corn kernels without hull or germ. They are usually bought in tins, and make a much better texture for chili than whole sweetcorn does.

Serves: 4.
Prep time: 5 minutes.
Cooking: 8 hours on low.
Smart Points: 7

Ingredients:
- 2 cans of diced tomatoes
- 1 can of **hominy**
- 1 can of kidney beans
- ¼ cup of **sour cream**
- ¼ cup of **cheddar**
- 4 squares of dark chocolate
- 2 tablespoons of chili powder
- 2 tablespoons of cilantro
- 1 teaspoon of cumin
- salt and pepper

Directions:
1. Mix all the ingredients in the slow cooker.
2. Cook on a low for 8 hours.

<u>**Nutritional values per serving**</u>: *KCAL: 171; net C 23g; P 12g; F 6.5g. Serve with crusty bread.*

2. Santa Fe Black Beans.

Black beans are highly nutritious bean with a very mild taste that takes on a lot of the flavors around it. This dish makes a roughly stewed black bean, but you can always mash, fry and re-fry the beans.

Serves: 7.
Prep time: 5 minutes.
Cooking: 8 hours on low.
Smart Points: 7

Ingredients:
- 1lb of dry black beans
- 3 cups of vegetable bouillon
- 2 cups of diced onion
- 1 cup of **queso fresco**
- 1 chopped chipotle chile
- ½ cup of fresh cilantro, chopped
- 2 tablespoons of minced garlic
- 1 tablespoon of lime juice
- salt and pepper

Directions:
1. Mix all the ingredients except for the queso fresco in a slow cooker.
2. Cook on a low pressure for 8 hours.
3. Add the queso fresco and pour on top.

Nutritional values per serving: KCAL: 130; net C 26g; P 20g; F 9g. Serve with fresh cilantro and cornbread.

3. Chicken And Chickpea Tagine.

Not all bean recipes are vegetarian. There are many wonderful combinations of meats and beans, such as with this delightful tagine.

Serves: 8.
Prep time: 20 minutes.
Cooking: 8 hours on low.
Smart Points: 8
Ingredients:
- 8 chicken thighs
- 2.5 cups of chopped red onion
- 2 cans of chickpeas
- 1 cup of chicken stock
- spicy Moroccan herb mix
- 2 tablespoons of **honey**
- salt and pepper

Directions:
1. Mix all ingredients in the slow cooker.
2. Cook on a low for 8 hours.

Nutritional values per serving: *KCAL: 255; net C 26.5g; P 22g; F 7g. Serve with lemon wedges for extra seasoning.*

4. White Bean And Smoked Ham Soup.

Another bean recipe that uses meat as a flavor enhancer, this recipe is a new take on pea and ham soup. The white beans absorb more flavor and provides more bite than peas do, making a delightful change.

Serves: 8.
Prep time: 5 minutes.
Cooking: 8 hours on low.
Smart Points: 7
Ingredients:
- 2lbs of smoked ham, diced
- 1lb of dried white beans
- 4 cups of chicken stock
- 1 cup of chopped onion
- 1 cup of chopped celery
- 1 cup of chopped carrot
- 3 tablespoons of minced garlic
- Herb mix
- salt and pepper

Directions:
1. Mix all ingredients in slow cooker.
2. Cook on a low for 8 hours.

Nutritional values per serving: *KCAL: 260; net C 26g; P 20g; F 5g. Serve with fresh crusty bread.*

5. Cincinnati Chili.

This variant on chili from, you guessed it, Cincinnati, is much warmer thanks to the addition of cinnamon and other Eastern spices.

Serves: 8.
Prep time: 5 minutes.
Cooking: 8 hours on low.
Smart Points: 8

Ingredients:
- 2.5lbs of mince meat
- 3 cans of red kidney beans
- 2 cans of chopped tomatoes
- 2 tablespoons of eastern spice mix
- 1 tablespoon of warm Christmas spice mix, including cinnamon and nutmeg
- 1 tablespoon of minced garlic
- salt and pepper

Directions:
1. Mix all the ingredients in the slow cooker.
2. Cook on a low for 8 hours.

Nutritional values per serving: KCAL: 276; net C 32g; P g26.5; F 6g.
Serve over spaghetti, the traditional way.

6. Black Bean And Sweet Potato Chili.

This black bean vegetarian chili swaps some of the traditional tomatoes for chopped sweet potato, adding a creamier texture and sweeter edge that goes very well with the black beans.

Serves: 4.
Prep time: 5 minutes.
Cooking: 8 hours on low.
Smart Points: 6
Ingredients:
- 3 cans of black beans
- 1 can of chopped tomato
- 1 cup of diced sweet potato
- 1 cup of diced onion
- ¼ cup fresh cilantro, chopped
- ¼ cup of **sour cream** or alternative
- 1 tablespoon of chili paste
- 1 tablespoon of minced garlic
- 1 tablespoon of cumin
- salt and pepper

Directions:
1. Mix all ingredients in slow cooker.
2. Cook on low for 8 hours.

<u>*Nutritional values per serving*</u>: *KCAL: 165; net C 20g; P 14g; F 6g. Serve over rice with extra herbs as garnish.*

7. White Lime Tofu Chili.

All chili benefits from some sour cream or yoghurt, but this vegetarian one focuses on white beans, yoghurt, and lime to bring out a unique taste.

Serves: 6.
Prep time: 5 minutes.
Cooking: 8 hours on low.
Smart Points: 6

Ingredients:
- 1.5lbs of firm silken **tofu**, cubed and fried
- 2 cans of white beans
- 2 cups of bouillon
- 1.5 cup of chopped onion
- ½ cup of **yoghurt** or alternative
- 3 tablespoon of lime juice
- 2 tablespoons of Tabasco sauce
- 2 tablespoons of minced garlic
- salt and pepper

Directions:
1. Mix all the ingredients in the slow cooker.
2. Cook on a low for 8 hours.

Nutritional values per serving: *KCAL: 198; net C 14g; P 25g; F 4g.*
Serve with corn bread.

8. Black Bean Soup.

This traditional soup recipe is hearty, warm and just perfect for a cold day.

Serves: 6.
Prep time: 5 minutes.
Cooking: 8 hours on low.
Smart Points: 7
Ingredients:
- 1lb of dry black beans
- 4 cups of bouillon
- 2 cups of chopped onion
- 1 cup of water
- ¼ cup of fresh cilantro
- 2 tablespoons of lime juice
- 1 tablespoon of chili paste
- Herb mix
- 3 bay leaves
- salt and pepper

Directions:
1. Mix all ingredients in the slow cooker.
2. Cook on a low pressure for 8 hours.

<u>Nutritional values per serving</u>: *KCAL: 286; net C 31g; P 17g; F 2g. Serve with sour cream or an alternative.*

Conclusion

Beyond all reasonable doubts, it is indisputably clear that the use of a crock pot is time-saving and easy to make a wide variety of healthy meals in order to suit your everyday meals, as it is vividly painted in this book. Hope this book has provided you with the resources you need to know about Weight Watchers Program and Crock Pot using. Hope you have found your favorite dishes for your Weight Watchers life. Best wishes!

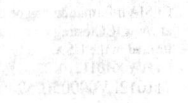

CPSIA information can be obtained
at www.ICGtesting.com
Printed in the USA
LVHW061011210222
711612LV00005B/59

9 781637 839294